CONFESSIONS OF A DEPRESSION SURVIVOR

NISHTHA SINGHAL

For

Madhu Juneja, Dr. Puneet Dwevedi, Aarti Rustagi, Tanvi Kaur, Dr. Prasan Deep Rath

Asha & Indra Kumar Singhal, Dr. Noopur & Dr. Ambuj Sud

Vikas, Aakriti, Archana & Mohan Deepak

Charu Mittal, Prerna Sinha, Shourie Anand Singh

Sanjivini Society for Mental Health, New Delhi

Minds Matter, Gurugram

I am blessed to have such a support system. Words are not enough to thank you all.

Contents

Preface

Trigger warning:

It is my humble request that if you are feeling low right now, please keep this book away for later so you are not triggered further. The book is written from a place of strength, but it can serve as a reminder of your struggle and unsettle you, though the idea is to offer you hope.

> *She lives, she suffers*
> *She battles, she wins*
> *She falls, she gets up*
> *She falls again, she gets up again*
> *She hopes, she shares hope*
> *With someone like her.*

Frankly, I don't know if you are someone like me. I am writing this book to share my learnings and insights from living with chronic mental illness and the related physical ailments. There is definitely someone out there that can help you. I can promise that you are not alone. No matter how unique your suffering, you can overcome it. That's my belief.

When I started suffering, there was no diagnosis. I had no vantage point, I was fearful. I didn't know which battle I was fighting. It wasn't cancer, brain tumour, death of a loved one, car accident, abduction, rape or any other catastrophe that as a teenager I had heard of. All I knew was I was suffering as much, if not more, than people encountered with one of the above. Then why wasn't I getting help? Why weren't people lining up to see me and say they're there for me. I was so miserable I wanted to die but nobody knew it and I didn't have the language to tell them.

What I was going through was as life threatening, if not more, than someone battling terminal physical illness. The latter desperately wants to live. I too had the will to live but along with it, I had the strongest urge to end it all in one stroke of self harm. It was scary. It was lonely. I didn't have a doctor to deliver the bad news to me or to my loved ones. I had to be the one to do it.

There are so many people out there whose suffering is so unique that they don't have access to a commonly understood vocabulary in which to explain it to themselves, and to their loved ones. You have to connect the dots. And what emerges will not be the same as anyone out there, right?

So, who is someone like you? Or someone like me? If you are trying to connect the dots of your suffering and learning how to live your life with that shape of suffering, I am someone like you, and you are someone like me.

Don't feel alone because there are so many that feel alone like you, so can you really be alone? I always heard there is light at the end of the tunnel. I used to think my tunnel was different and would forever remain dark. It was different, yes, but only because every tunnel is unique. But there is light at the end of 'every' tunnel. I invite you to read some notes I have put together at various points through my journey with illness and treatment. I am merely sharing my experience and through that, prescribing hope to you, nothing more, nothing less. If at any point it seems like I am prescribing a cure, a solution, or giving medical advice, please read it as a note to myself, not to you. Every patient has a different prognosis. Since our journeys are unique, the specific techniques and ideas that worked for me, might not work for you. Be in touch with your therapist and doctor and be true to your treatment, rather than take suggestions from those who don't understand your condition and your coping.

If you want to share your journey or that of someone you care about, write to me. If you wish to seek treatment, I will provide references of skilled and sincere practitioners. The first person or professional you reach out to may or may not be the right fit, but don't lose hope. Try talking to them about your difficulty with them before you move to someone else.

If you like the book, please pass it on or gift a copy. Spread and share the hope!

Nishtha Singhal

2024

Gurugram, India

Acknowledgements

I want to thank the illness and the prognosis for lending itself to this book. Depression emerged as my muse for cultivating a language of suffering, surviving, coping and hoping. With depression, I have grown up a bit. There is more growing up to be done.

I want to thank this book for giving me the opportunity to revisit some parts of my journey that needed revisiting and for helping me find closure in some areas that must reach a conclusion now.

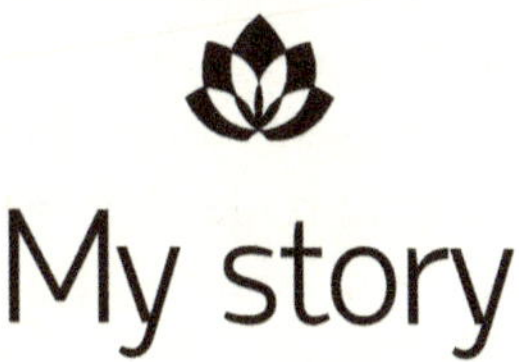

CHAPTER ONE

My story

I was born in Bathinda, Punjab in 1986. With little recollection of life's first 5 years, I start my story from my fifth birthday when I moved to Lagos with my parents and elder sister. The 3.25 years spent there make for the best period of my life, though I am told I used to be sick and crying often back then as well. All I remember is sheer bliss of childhood, family, friends, trips to the beach, pot lucks, Christmas and New Year parties. I never really got over the dreamy and perfect perception of my childhood in Nigeria.

We returned to India when I was 8. We now know that I did not take this transition well, emotionally. I went to school (graduated 2004) and college (graduated 2007) in New Delhi. By 2001, something had started going seriously wrong but nobody could tell exactly what. All the symptoms of clinical depression were there but all the treatment was targeted at the physical symptoms. Mental illness was not even on the family doctor's mind and that of the various specialists I went to for several recurring issues with physical health. Nobody suspected mental illness until 2003 when a homeopath hinted at it. We rubbished it proclaiming that the sadness stemmed from a general absence of well-being owing to falling sick very frequently and being sensitive emotionally.

Then in 2005, in second year of college, an online checklist I encountered was enough to convince me I had depression. I saw a psychiatrist. I was told you have had depression for a long time now; it has progressed and you need medication. I heard him out but protested that I will get sucked into a web of drugs that were notorious for being addictive. I agreed to try counselling; it didn't seem all that outlandish in 2005. Unluckily, I got no results from that. Not once did I question my denial to take medicines, always hoping that I was mentally well and it was just my immunity that needed work. I kept fooling myself that there was no monster, till July 2, 2007, when it let itself out. There was no denying it anymore.

It was day two at my first job after graduation, a coveted role at a business consulting firm in Gurugram. It was a hectic day with back to back orientation sessions. I could hear everything, but was registering nothing. At lunch, I had difficulty placing my order. Finally when I did order, by the time the food arrived, I didn't remember what I had ordered. Wanting to disappear rather than be seen for the difficult time I was having and the confusion I would create, I made no effort to find my order and went hungry. Seated in a conference room with the other new hires, I retreated into a nightmare. I don't remember if I stayed till end of day or how I managed to get back home. All I remember is hitting the bed on getting home and tearing into cries for help. The very next day, I was in the office of one of the most experienced psychiatrists in New Delhi at the time, no longer averse to medication, and scared like hell that it was too late already.

Major depressive disorder, without a diagnosed cause in my case, had tied my mind up in knots. These knots had become further complicated with ignorance and denial of the condition for six years since I first started feeling the symptoms. I had been inspiring sadness into my mind, endlessly. It soon started getting worse and started eating into my family and friends' strength to support me. In the grip of trauma by now, numbed and merely drifting in time and space, we had not experienced anything of this magnitude before. Finding any meaning in the situation seemed beyond us.

Till mid-2008, my condition did not respond well to treatment. I was on heavy medication and on some sort of psychotherapy as well, but I kept worsening. Disillusioned, I abruptly quit medication and psychotherapy. I have never since spoken to these practitioners. I ghosted them and drifted into a phase where I declared to family and friends that I am OK, there is no illness and no treatment required. I decided I will fix myself by myself and there was nothing to be said or done about it. I indulged myself in the fancy that I was all powerful. I created a wall nobody could breach.

This ended in a breakdown in May 2009, when I got to the point of wanting to end it all and became suicidal, but I really wanted to live as well. For one last chance at life, on May 14, 2009, I dialed the suicide helpline of Sanjivini, and a female voice answered, and heard me out like nobody had ever heard me out before. Somehow, in her voice, I found that there was hope for me after all. She talked me into committing that I will see a psychiatrist immediately. I noted the details of the psychiatrist, took an appointment and met him the very next day. Later that week, I met her.

She was to be my counsellor. The wheels of me returning to life were set in motion then, and have been turning since.

Sanjivini Society for Mental Health became life's way of telling me that there is somebody who understands the mess I am in, even if I don't understand it. I realised I wasn't alone, that my loved ones want to help me but I was pushing them away. My counsellor and psychiatrist did not dismiss me when I howled in emotional trauma, and did not get overwhelmed by my pain either. Gradually, they prepared me for a journey of healing, recognizing and appreciating my desire to get better.

Within a few weeks, I discovered I was ANA positive and had borderline lupus. This meant I could get lupus in future. One of the top rheumatologists of India diagnosed me with undifferentiated connective tissue disease (UCTD), an auto immune condition. I had persistent low grade fever, aches in the small joints, and fatigue. There was no telling if the depression had brought this on or I had it all along, even as a child. With this diagnosis, I was in for a lifelong dependence on an immuno-suppressant drug called HCQS (made infamous during the COVID 19 pandemic) to protect my organs from my own immune system. I was also put on a blood thinner to protect my heart.

Though I was hearing of this illness and its treatment for the first time and was now fighting one more battle, the UCTD diagnosis brought more relief than despair, at least initially. There was science behind what I was going through and why I was suffering so much. So what if the diagnosis was so unclear; I was being treated by the best. The best part was there were safe medicines available and accurate tests. I was not going to suffer endlessly once I decided that the illnesses can be confronted, understood, tackled and conquered. I started believing I was never going to give up again. It was just a matter of following the doctor's advice religiously.

Soon, the treatment got too much for me. I was drained from all the medication and confused about the prognosis, more so of the UCTD than the depression. I was fighting the UCTD more in my mind than in my body. My perception of being sick was far more heightened than the actual sickness in my body. Though I was lucky to have the love of family and friends, sadly, I was too unwell to receive their help and care, and kept rejecting them. I isolated myself. I was trying to fight it all by myself and shutting out the people in my life who could share my burden. This was the first challenge my counsellor and psychiatrist helped me with. They gradually guided me back to a position where I could feel connected to my loved ones.

This time, I was being treated by health professionals I felt comfortable sharing every detail of my suffering and coping with. Their professionalism, care and understanding was of a much higher standard than had been my experience previously. My family and friends also embraced my challenges as their own and created the space in which my treatment could progress in the right direction. They pushed limits and stretched all they could, to make sure the journey continued. We worked as a team, all devoted to the cause of helping me feel healed.

The pace of the healing was frustratingly slow. I would keep falling behind, and cursing myself for the failures. With repeated disappointments and failure of my efforts to feel better, and the end of the tunnel seeming to move farther and farther, I was tempted to give up many times, but somehow, I always kept going back to my counsellor, psychiatrist, and rheumatologist for review, medicine titrations, and tests. This was because I hoped it would get easier, and with the trust I had developed in my medical team, I knew I had to try to find that way and their intervention would enable me to do just that. Every time I met my counsellor and psychiatrist, they showed me how far I had come, while I was always showing them how much more distance I had left to cover. I would even start crying in my rheumatologist's office and waiting room, looking at all the other patients who were at least thrice my age. I felt so lonely there. What was I doing fighting arthritis at this age, when I should be studying or working. I would have a pity party ever so often back then. The concern of my future and comparison with contemporaries made me undermine my progress, but with the continuous intervention of my counsellor and psychiatrist, and reassurances from my loved ones, I was able to accept the journey and appreciate my efforts. It was a constant struggle to maintain this attitude, but there was no other way to approach the journey.

Over the next year or so, I grew from strength to strength but not without several setbacks. I stumbled constantly, giving in to the tiredness of living with two chronic illnesses. After every fall, I trusted myself again, and started walking by myself. There was no freedom from the illness, but a sense of freedom from its power to consume my will to carry on. So empowered and supported compared to the pathetic state of 2007, in October 2010, I went on to get a diploma in Montessori Method of Early Childhood Education and even worked as co-class teacher in a class of toddlers for a month before I had to quit because I got exhausted from the effort. I tried again the following year. I enrolled for the two year Masters in English Literature at Jawaharlal Nehru University, completed it, and worked in the Communications Team for a little less than a year at a major grant-making organisation in the sustainable energy space. All this while, I was fighting the illnesses and sincerely pursuing my treatment. For two years, I drove 10 kms each way to JNU for classes. I even moved to an apartment at a stone's throw from my office, and lived the dream of sharing an apartment with best friends. The medical team helped me make tweaks that would allow me to sustain my study and work schedules. Stepping out and living life, although still in the shadow of chronic illness, was helping me more than it was demanding from me. But, soon, the difficulty started piling up. I revolted so much, always wanting to give up and asking why it was so hard, but I am glad I stayed in the mainstream lane of life for as long as I did. In mid-2014, I had to return to life in the recovery lane.

By now, the constant struggle to manage the symptoms of depression and UCTD and the side effects of all the medication for both conditions had drained me out completely. (Weight gain, dry skin, dry mouth, getting startled easily, tremors, restless leg syndrome, increased appetite, the list is endless and honestly, there was no respite ever from the side effects. They only got compounded; I have gotten used to them now. They never do go away.) I started leaning endlessly on my support systems and drifted into learned helplessness, i.e. I started seeing being unwell as comfortable. I started sabotaging my own recovery by not stepping out of this comfort zone and demanding that others take care of me. I believed I was too tired to carry on by myself, and that all my reservoirs were empty. I started resenting having to take care of myself.

Quitting the job was the best decision I took. I wanted to focus on treatment. My medical team was still with me, as were my family and friends, although I thought I had let them all down. In a year's time, I progressed to a point where I was seen to be ready for working with a psychotherapist for behavioral and cognitive work. The thought patterns that were still maintaining my depression were arresting healing and sabotaging my own efforts to progress. In July 2015, I transitioned from counselling to psychotherapy. Counselling had achieved its purpose of sustaining me to the point where I was ready to attack the illness at its roots.

With the addition of psychotherapy into my treatment, I started developing an awareness of my 'self' and reconnecting with 'Nishtha' independent of the illness. Life's demands and realities still seemed out of bounds, but I knew that with healing, I would be able to become stronger than the illness, and ultimately reach the point where I could tackle these demands and realities. Slowly, I could see that I was less a victim than I felt I was. I started recognizing my thinking patterns, my limiting beliefs and my insecurities. At the same time, I began to gradually understand that I also possessed defenses, capabilities and strengths against the negative currents that depression launches. I started cultivating them as tools against the depression. I started attacking guilt, shame, self-pity, and self-loathing. I learnt to constantly remind myself to love myself, respect my capacities, reconsider my fears and expectations. I acquired a language to talk about my thoughts and resulting feelings, and picked up skills to check my cognitive distortions.

I was making gains but my sense of control over my mind was still weak. It took infinitely longer than I would have liked. Nothing could have prepared me for the shockingly slow pace of my healing even after starting psychotherapy. I incessantly questioned the faith that I would get better. I would keep counting the years I had lost already, and compared myself to all those who had not found themselves caught in the tide of this disorder. Nothing could console me. I grew frustrated with the treatment, and I demanded of my healers to put a time frame on the process. I was turning 30 and still waiting for life to begin. I would threaten my loved ones with the possibility that I might not want to carry on with life. Every now and then, the tiredness from the sluggish pace of my healing would threaten to end everything. But the desire to get better always got the better of these rock-bottom episodes. I realized there was no waiting to be done; the living had to start in the here and now, along with the illness and exhaustion. In therapy, I benefitted immensely and still do. My first book, *Psychotherapy for Depression: Personal Essays by a Survivor* presents insights from my psychotherapy from 2015-2022.

Bit by bit, my healing progressed. The end of the tunnel became visible. Thought patterns improved. Self sabotaging behavior gave way to self-enabling voices in my head. No, the movement is not always in the right direction...sometimes the circuits back fire and the efforts flow back into the wrong direction, but the tide turns again. The journey continues, without a destination to arrive at. Life is now made up of moments in which I feel there has been progress and healing.

In early 2024, at 37, I approach my life with more strength than pity, more like a challenger than a challenged one, more like a patient than a victim. I see a method to my suffering now. I indulge less and less in unhealthy comparisons with people whose journey has been different than mine, with or without mental illness. At the same time, I appreciate the multifarious struggles that every human being faces and do not undermine their suffering. I don't think that I am the odd one out; even though I feel so every now and then.

It has taken very long to get here. I continue to need treatment, support and reassurance. The best part is that my medical team, family and friends continue to be by my side. More importantly, I draw support from them in more constructive and healthier ways than earlier. Today, I am empowered enough to share my journey and hope that more and more people will believe that depression does not have to end in suicide. I won't lie; I tried thrice to end it all between 2007 and 2017 but am still here. My actions were more about a desire to feel less pain rather than a desire to not live. I wanted to get better, not cease to exist, but I was helpless that I wasn't getting better. I am glad I did not succeed in ending it all. Unfortunately, many people succeed in one of their attempts. Nobody ever "commits" suicide; it is always an "attempt," because actually their act of harming themselves is an attempt to end their pain, not their life.

CHAPTER TWO

Taking life one day at a time

Chronic illness swallowed up the sense of fitness and health. I not only lost access to it, but all imagination of it disappeared from my psyche. I forgot what it felt like to not be sick. Twenty-four seven, 365 days a year, I felt how I imagined a pregnant woman must feel like. Accepting the new normal has been a long battle. Not even medication can help with this emotional pain of chronic illness. This is like coping with death of an earlier version of yourself, which had an experience of wholesomeness of mind and body. A part of you has succumbed to the illness. You grieve it but you also live for the part that's still alive. This grief tugs at your heart's strings strongly but you disengage from it so you can live and attach with other less painful areas in life. This requires distractions like social engagements, volunteering etc. to create positive currents or a different layer of your life which takes the focus away from suffering to living. That's your distraction, your faking it till you make it. It might seem like just surviving and not living. I thought I am barely surviving while others get to live a full life. I realised soon enough that everyone was barely surviving, one way or another. Living and surviving are two sides of the same coin.

There are days when I am so angry at my illness that I want to end my life so I can be free of the experience of living with illness. Sinking to the point of suicidal ideation several times has been a dark reality of my experience of suffering long-term with depression. But, with treatment, time and the consistent support of loved ones, I am empowered to a point where now, I patiently wait for this anger to pass. I can pull myself out and distract myself from the ideas of self-harm and immerse my mind and body in activities that have come to bring relief over the years. It could be a movie or coffee outing with my husband, going to the salon, calling up my mom, sister or best friend and crying my lungs out, talking to my therapist on the phone, reporting to the psychiatrist for a timely intervention in terms of medication, listening to songs that speak to me, having F.R.I.E.N.D.S or BBT going in the background for emotional support, Maggi noodles, relaxing while crying to yog nidra or progressive muscle relaxation audios, binge crocheting with YouTube videos of my favourite makers like Sarah Jayne or Melanie Ham, coloring in my adult coloring book, writing to my diary, reading the notes from my therapy sessions, organizing or decorating my room, picking out clothes to donate from my wardrobe, chucking stuff in the trashcan, cooking pasta in pesto sauce with basil leaves from my own plant, ordering chocolate cake, showering with grapefruit shower cream...something or the other always ends up holding me in a warm embrace of self-care...and reminding me that I do want to carry on still...and the anger-filled day passes. I rest for a few days to overcome the impact, and then rise again to take one day at a time.

And then there are the days when I am not angry enough to get suicidal but struggling nonetheless...engaging with the source of my aches and pains, asking questions about the prognosis, seeking clarity about treatment, harboring hope about complete recovery, making guesses about causes, building scenarios and plans about better managing the illness, negotiating with reality and schemes in my head...all the time insisting on more answers...not letting go of the desire to feel better and free of sickness.

And then there are the rest of the days. These are the days when I am feeling together enough to want to continue. They don't last for long but they always come back. So, I hang in here waiting for them. And then I remember to mark them in my mind as the days worth living for. I remember them. I record them and count them as my blessings. Although I complain a lot, because it is so tough to live this life, on days when the fog is not so dense, I can see silver linings in the clouds of illness surrounding me. It has taken more than 15 years to not feel alone and different in this world, but it has been the most important victory of my journey. My husband, mother, father and sister, and my extended family through these four; my close friends; my body; and my counselor, psychiatrist, psychotherapist and rheumatologist have walked by my side for real or in spirit, every single day, no matter what my strengths that day. I have learnt over the years to internalise their support and holding, rather than to seek them out each time I feel the need. When I do seek them out, they are there for me, whatever their strengths that day.

CHAPTER THREE

Doing what makes me happy

What does it mean to do what makes you happy?

You do not have to think hard about what makes you happy. Only the thing that makes you happy without riders attached is the answer to this question. That means, you don't have to worry about doing that thing well, doing that thing all the time, doing that thing regularly, doing that thing in a particular way...it just has to be something that makes you happy in that moment, whether or not you enjoy doing it as a hobby, profession, pastime, creative outlet etc. You do not have to define these things based on categories that may work for others. The categories of others and the world at large, may or may not work for you.

Your definition of happiness is unique to you. What makes you happy may just be a fancy you enjoy indulging in. It may be an un-doing kind of thing, like cleaning something, throwing away stuff you don't need, scribbling with a gel-pen, tearing paper, getting hands dirty in clay or even sand. The thing that makes you happy doesn't even have to be a thing. It can be a non-thing, like taking a nap, or sitting on a park bench while others are going about their daily exercise, evening walk, whatever.

We form an association of comfort, stress release and, sense of recovery with certain things, and when we are overwhelmed, they soothe us through instant gratification. There is no shame in using things for self-soothing. For example, some of the things that have started working for me after years of struggling to achieve a certain 'happy' effect are:

i. watching sitcoms from the 90s

ii. colouring

iii. crocheting

iv. undoing my crochet project and creating something finer

v. plucking basil leaves from my balcony and making pesto

vi. painting on loose sheets of paper or in a notebook without a design in mind

vii. watching videos of the babies in the family

viii. retail therapy at the malls (within a budget), followed by coffee and snack

One must remember that in making yourself happy for some time, you will not be able to overcome pain and sadness, or memories associated with a loss. It only means that in those moments you will be distracted from (rather than feel overwhelmed by) these emotions. That is pleasure and that is what 'do what makes you happy' means to me. Don't have too many expectations from the activity, only then it will allow you few moments of happiness. And while doing the activity, try to be mindful of the activity itself, not what it is making you feel. When I stopped trying to make them work, I started experiencing pleasure in doing these activities. It took me many years to realise this. Then again, they don't work all the time. As long as you keep the faith and don't abandon them for good, they will unleash a whole lot of happiness every now and then. The idea is to gather such moments over a period of time, so that your mind starts believing that happiness is a possible state, even for you. This will start taking away from the strength of the depression and the power it has over your being.

CHAPTER FOUR

Listening to myself, not the depression

The victimhood feeling, of something tragic having happened to me, became constant over the years. I couldn't shake off the feeling of 'my life has been snatched away from me due to illness.' I was constantly resenting this victim identity but also holding onto it, not able to let go. The depression was feeding on my victim identity and strengthening it at the same time. This was learned helplessness. The depression was making me feel like a victim, to seek sympathy and care and lean on caregivers even when I didn't need to. The anger and frustration around the illness was maintaining and worsening it. I started feeling weak and that I cannot take care of myself. I lost touch with the part of myself that was fighting the depression and trying to rebuild life. I started operating inside a cocoon. I stopped challenging myself or my limits. I believed that I cannot help myself; someone has to rescue me. I was surrendering my power to the depression. This was exacerbated by the fibromyalgia. I was always in pain and so drained of energy that I didn't feel up to doing anything, or interested in doing anything, leave alone exercising to counter the depression. Brushing my teeth, showering and leaving my room, was all I could achieve in the entire day and was still drained and exhausted by the effort, as if I didn't have a moment to breathe and pause all day...as if on a treadmill twenty four seven. In fact, it was the mind which was on a treadmill all day, not me. In such a scenario, the medicines could do little to help me. In a way, my depression was now resisting treatment. I needed to break out of this cycle.

Over several years in therapy, I started seeing myself as separate from the depression. No matter how feeble and transient, there was always a voice present in me that knew better than to believe the depression's chatter. That voice struggled to make its presence felt, but my therapist made me see that part of Nishtha. Even if only momentarily and sometimes only for me to dismiss her immediately as hardly any good, I started meeting that Nishtha in my therapy sessions. At first, she was weak and I was unable to access her. I had to strengthen her voice and make her feel 'seen' and 'heard', especially when the depression was trying to drown her. The moment I would side with her, the depression would get threatened. This voice had two parts to her - Nishtha, the child and Nishtha, the adult.

Depression is not my true self, but a self-fulfiling distortion of my true self. I am the whole truth. My dreams, my memories, my achievements, my strengths, my experiences...they are all intact inside me, despite years of pain piled over them. I cannot lose my self to an illness, no matter how hijacked and overpowered by it I feel. The illness has created an illusion of suffering and buried me under layers of pain. Even after some of that pain has been addressed or healed, the illusion remains. The depression uses my perception of this pain to take my power away, define how I think, what I say, and most importantly make choices for me. It justifies all my tantrums and my inertia, so that I continue to nurture the helplessness inside me. It masquerades as a needy weak self, trying to mimic my inner child and make me reject her. It is like throwing the baby with the bath water. However, I have learnt to identify the depression and label it as 'not me'.

I started seeing the child in me that was feeling safe in the comfort zone of being cared for and rescued by others. I acknowledged her need and slowly guided her into a space of saying 'no' to the depression, rather than fusing with the depression's own voice. I unlearned the learned helplessness by first befriending the child Nishtha, then slowly nudging her to a healthier behavior. I imagined her to be a reservoir of my life's experiences, especially the difficult ones. She needed reassurance because she was afraid and insecure about life outside the comfort zone. She didn't know how to express this fear, so she was acting out through tantrums and resistance to push her limits. I slowed down the recovery process to accommodate her, to hug her and not rush her, but also to gently challenge her belief that stepping out would be catastrophic. I had to parent her by not always giving in to her terms but also not discounting her needs. I took ownership of her tantrums as my own, rather than alienating her and labeling her childish. I identified with the child Nishtha as much as I wanted to associate with the adult Nishtha. Slowly, both started working together because both wanted to grow, rather than languish in the darkness. I learnt there was nothing to be ashamed and guilty about. I had one duty towards both of them, to love them and protect them. But first, I had to accept them and listen to them without judgement.

This is how I distinguished my own voice amidst the depression's chatter. The struggle was to shift my mind's radio station from the depression to the real me. The controls of my mind were so feeble and worn out from the depression, that the knob always tended to tilt to the depression side. Such was the pull of the monster that had been created from an imbalance in the hormones. I had to practise keeping that knob in place, precariously hanging on to it with awareness, reminders and guidance. It took a lot of time to get that grip. But I heard my voice finally.

Unlike the depression, my voice offers me my power, rather than taking over from me. I now have a mechanism to comfort and console myself by myself, challenge the negative spiral and ultimately, feel better by myself. I no longer depend on the therapist for every bad day or whenever I slip from the baseline. Staying afloat does not require intervention from my doctor. I get to a point of drowning but still come back up for air and get stable. I do feel like a victim but I also counter that feeling with the right thought about why I am feeling that way. I can explain this with a simple example.

If I feel I am sinking into a low, I want to lie down and hide in bed, rather than to tackle it in an active manner. The voice of Nishtha will warn me that I'm giving in to the depression's demand to hit the bed, but I give in anyway and lie down. But sometimes, I am able to re-hear Nishtha and create space in my mind to really listen to her and understand her suggestion. She is not dismissing how tired I am of fighting, how sad I am in this moment and how desperately I want to shut down the barrage of thoughts that are threatening my very will to carry on. She is barely reminding me to consider, "Is there another way to deal with this?" She is not undermining my pain, but merely showing me that if I could recalibrate my pain perception right now, would I be able to attempt a slightly better threshold? Sometimes, I shoot her down and feel if I don't do so, I will spiral and hit rock bottom. I drown her voice in the pain and don't even register the reminder. It's almost like she spoke only after I already hit the bed, or she probably didn't speak at all. The truth is, she spoke, but I couldn't hear her. She got drowned. But sometimes I hear her.

These are the signs of healing. The healthier side of me never died, but with healing, I have been able to hear her more often than not.

CHAPTER FIVE

Appreciating mental fog, rest, and progress

Every day I would struggle with the thought of 'Am I doing enough to keep the depression at bay, and secure my future from it?' My mind would allow a constant chatter of what I 'should' be doing right now, rather than recalling what I have already 'done' today. The 'should' statement made my head and heart heavier and heavier, to the extent that I would not be able to remember what part of the day I am in, which is going to be my next meal, and what day of the week it is. Complete disorientation. Why? Because I was trying to push myself to create a certain kind of day, that is productive, includes exercise, right eating, staying out of bed...and so on. This became an agenda to torture myself, rather than to deal with the illness. This is how I experienced mental fog. It was a trap that I got into, living with the illness for so long.

The thought of wanting to fight the depression and emerge healed had become so powerful that it consumed all my energy, which I needed to create positive sustained action towards actually healing. Pushing too hard was not helping me, rather harming me. There was no shortcut to emerging out of a tunnel. Balance of consistent effort and sustained energy in the right direction was a skill I acquired with therapy and practise. When I have mental fog, I try to be kind to myself. I let my mind be. This is the time it is asking for space. It is overstimulated by the 'should' thoughts and is feeling burdened. Instead of being kind to it, I am making it feel like it ought to perform better, remember better, and make my body move better, so that the day is a certain way, which is how I will beat the depression, and there is no other way apparently.

It takes me a very long time to recover from a bout of physical sickness like viral fever, food poisoning, seasonal flu or allergies. With the depression and the auto immune condition gripping the mind and body in an obnoxious cycle of losing energy and heightened pain perception, I take forever to bounce back. Rest is the only answer. But resting is very hard for me because my mind keeps nagging me with the worry that I am not doing something I could or should be doing. I am depleted in energy, spirit and any semblance of motivation to do anything, but my mind, instead of allowing me to rest, keeps asking me what could and should I be doing but am not doing. I try to watch something on Netflix, I try to lie down, I try to clean a bit, I try to write...but the mind does not say even once that what you are doing is alright, but reminds me that you could and should be doing something else, something more productive, whatever 'more' means.

I feel extremely unproductive and almost worthless for needing so much rest, and not being able to 'perform' as a 'normal' individual who has taken a few sick days. The sick days are never few in my case. It takes ages to recover my strength. I know that every time I get derailed by physical sickness, and I become dysfunctional, I bounce back in several days to some semblance of well-being and routine. But, tiding over these days is very unsettling. I continue to put up with the chatter, hoping and praying that it will pass in a few days and I will feel better.

For years on end, I suffered this cycle of shame. Only recently, I have come to accept that this is what it is like and this is what it is going to be like. I can only work when I really can. I let myself rest for as long as I need to. I no longer allow physical sickness to make me feel worse about myself. I remember that I deserve to rest when I need it. It doesn't mean I have stopped or become unproductive on purpose; it just means I am resting till I can resume. When it seems that all I can manage is surviving and staying afloat somehow, I must remember that when 'doing mode' is so tough, 'being mode' is an achievement. While I feel under attack and find my body and mind giving up, I will have to rest and stop fighting the attack. I have to accept that it is passive, but it is needed and that there is no shame or laziness in this. I am not inadequate because of it. I should be compassionate to myself rather than expect results by pushing myself to achieve goals. This means accepting that with every few steps forward, I also come back a few steps and this is ok.

Therapy and time have helped me overcome self-defeating inner dialogues and respect myself as I am. With chronic sickness, it can be hard to feel worth anything more than a burden on loved ones. However, I remind myself my inherent worth, the reason we all take birth and exist in the life that we do, with the people that we are with. They are with me not because they can't leave, but because they want to be with me. The tide will turn; I will have good days. On those days, I will be able to function better.

I could not progress in certain journeys in life...such as being a lawyer, journalist, writer, teacher...roles that I dreamt I would play in life and prepared for in terms of obtaining degrees. I have not been able to cultivate a career or achieve financial independence. Further, I feel ill equipped to take the plunge into motherhood owing to my continuing health challenges. But I have enjoyed, and continue to enjoy many roles in life - daughter, sister, grandchild, niece, friend, aunt, wife, and also a language editor as and when health permits. I am also a self-taught crocheter. I have steadily grown in these roles, endured steep learning curves, and most importantly, experienced joy through living them and sharing life in this capacity with so many people in my life.

My suffering and my struggle to overcome it, has taught me that I have to appreciate and value all aspects of my life, at all times, not just the milestones on the linear path of life and success. No matter how much I lament and complain that all got snatched from me or I could have done and achieved so much more in life, and still can and should, deep inside, I still feel more privileged and blessed than most people on Earth. These statements (could, can, should) can unsettle me for a bit but soon enough, I remember my blessings and centre myself again in my 'one day at a time' mode. There's no telling where this mode will take me...perhaps one day I really 'would' surprise myself...now 'would' is not a harmful word to say to yourself.

When you are recovering, don't ignore the progress in any area. In some role, you may be stuck but in another, you are probably moving forward. Acknowledge and make use of what you already possess or achieve on a daily basis. Progress will not materialize in the order that you want. Some wheels are very deep in the quagmire and some are relatively less stuck. Any movement is healing, or is progress towards healing. Be grateful and attach yourself to your progress. Detach from the areas that are so deeply lost that they need more time and space. If you rush them, they will take longer. Let yourself arrive at them.

CHAPTER SIX

Struggling to exercise

Not being able to exercise had been the nagging pattern of my recovery journey. I have obsessed over not being able to do exactly that which will help me get better, as if exercise is a magic wand that if I could get a hold of, would become the undoing of all my problems in life. Every vein and nerve in me would reject exercise while I would try to reason with my mind and body that exercise will heal me faster and more holistically than any antidepressant or immunosuppressant ever can. In several of my therapy sessions, I have spoken about a vicious cycle of failure to exercise and not being able to reverse this, no matter what.

I have done yoga with a personal trainer; joined group classes for taichi, zumba, salsa, adult ballet; enroled for swimming and badminton at the club; worked out at gyms; tried walking with a friend and so on. Every time I would start, there would be hope of consistency, but overpowering that would be the aches and pains that came with any physical activity. My body was beyond stiff. Layers of visceral fat gained from years of medication and emotional eating shouted back at me, "You think you can reverse this, really?" "You think you can shake us out of the comfortable spaces we are lodged in, and in turn pump happy hormones? Think again." And think again I would. In fact I wouldn't stop thinking. I would obsess about how I want to cancel the session or class, how every part of my body is asking for a rest day, how the battle is so uphill I might as well give up. Year after year, I began working out and gave up...adding to the layers of fat around my internal organs, eating my feelings, staying up late at night further slowing the metabolism down, trying to think my worries out, solve my depression, only to have another lousy morning and afternoon, evening and night. This kept the weight on the rise.

I am still taking medication for depressive disorder and UCTD. I still indulge in emotional eating and have increased appetite and slow metabolism. From 55 in 2007, I am at 90 kgs in early 2024. Though I have made some strides over the years, I still struggle to exercise and check the weight gain. With all the excessive weight that collected around my organs, I developed disease in two other organs. I had to undergo surgery in one, and am on medication for the other. I am committed to make the lifestyle changes necessary for reversing these conditions but I struggle. I am trying and will not give up.

CHAPTER SEVEN

Circling back to self-pity

Every few months I get to a point where all I can talk about is how hard my life is. How hard it is to navigate every single aspect of my day.

"As your days are, so shall your strengths be."

This is something my counselor at Sanjivini wrote for me when I landed the first job since starting treatment. At the time, it felt like she was signaling to me to anticipate hard days ahead. Now I know she was signaling to me that I had what it would take to get past my days ahead.

Even today, days continue to be tough. On at least 30% of the hard days, my strengths match my days and I can breeze through. But 70% of the days are tough. After navigating every 100 or so such tough days, I emerge oh so bitter! Automatically, my system launches into a pity party where I complain to my partner, my mom, my best friends, sometimes to my dad and my sister too, and obviously to my therapist about

HOW I CAN'T CATCH A BREAK FROM THIS ILLNESS AND HOW IT CATCHES UP WITH ME DESPITE ALL MY EFFORTS AND HOW IT HAS DEFINED ALL MY ADULT LIFE AND I WANT TO ESCAPE IT ALL BECAUSE I AM SOOOO TIRED, I WOULD RATHER END IT ALL AND BE AT REST. WHY I THINK I SHOULD BE CUT SOME SLACK, WHY I FEEL I HAVE SUFFERED ENOUGH AND I AM NOW TIRED, WHY I JUST WANT IT ALL TO END AND I WANT TO ESCAPE...HOW I HAVE ENDURED EVERYTHING AND CAN'T OR DON'T WANT TO TAKE ANY MORE...

It feels petty to circle back to the same dark spot over and over, despite being in treatment for so long, surviving it all so many times over, writing about it, triumphing over it, but hitting the same dark spot again and again.

Since my diagnosis, this pity party took many forms...from suicidal attempts and ideation...to hating and cursing my caregivers...to hitting the headboard of the bed in distress...to trying to hurt myself by hitting the wall...wanting to trade the illness for cancer...cursing God...and more such ugliness. More recently, it comes in the form of an all-out crying spell with complete insight and awareness that I have come a long way and even the most gruesome tiredness and helplessness will not let me give up now, because time has shown that I will live through it, not die from it. It is now restricted to crying spells. Sometimes, I rescue myself even before tearing up. Beneath all the self-pity, there is inner strength. I just have to reach down to it, wading through the fatalism and bitterness.

CHAPTER EIGHT

Dreaming up another reality

Sometimes we conjure up a vision of our reality because it helps us to carry on in life because if we don't, life will be too unpalatable. It could be an imaginary friend, an obsessive love for a crush, a superhero attachment...or anything you feel very strongly about but which may not be apparent to anyone but you.

Preservation through building an alternate reality, not really true and what you wish reality to be like, is a coping mechanism for when the going gets tough. When we outgrow the difficult phase, the dream gets shattered. We feel embarrassed that we believed in something fantastical. How could we let ourselves get carried away by a vision and be indifferent to reality? How could we be in denial for so long?

Now is not the time to feel embarrassed but to thank yourself for dreaming up the vision that kept you alive. You created the circumstances to help yourself when all else seemed to go wrong in your life. Instead of putting yourself down for believeing in this fantasy, cherish it before you let it go forever. It anchored you, rescued you. Even if it created an illusion of wanting to live, it saved you from your demons of destruction. It held you, sustained you, and you emerged through the darkest cloud riding on it.

One such dream made me feel unusual optimism and strength about my future, even though I was sick and suicidal. This dream waited for me at the other end and made me want to navigate the tunnel. It made the suffering worth it. However, before I could make it to the other end, the dream shattered, and along with it, my will to go on. It was like being stranded in the middle of the ocean. The wind that had propelled my flight till then had suddenly disappeared from beneath my wings...or so I thought. I stopped trying to swim or fly; I let gravity take over. I was not only getting consumed in the darkness inside the tunnel, but also refusing that there was an end to walk towards, that the dream had disappeared, not the end. Without the dream, the end of the tunnel lost meaning for me. I had equated life with the dream. If the dream left, there was no living to be done. It was ugly. It was something everyone around me had dreaded because they knew I had mistaken the dream for my life but they could not force me to believe until I discovered it for myself.

Anyway, I did reimagine life without the dream and started navigating the tunnel again. Therapy and support of loved ones held me up every time I fell back into the fantasy and demanded the dream to come alive. They declined to let me go and let go of me. Giving up was not an option. This was the toughest and darkest stretch of the tunnel to navigate and took the longest to cross but this journey within my journey made me grow up by leaps and bounds and has prepared me for life's hardships.

Did I regret that I imagined the future a certain way? Do I regret that at one point, it disappeared? I did regret. I was so angry at myself for dreaming and at the dream for disappearing. But several years later, I can see that I needed to dream, and the dream needed to shatter. For me to create a dream life to walk towards and for it to shatter before I got to it, both had a purpose. I would have perished without the dream. And if it had forever been visible, I would not have fought hard enough to make it this far.

So, I cherish dreaming up another reality when my reality was unpalatable for living. I hope you will not be afraid to dream up a beautiful reality when you need to.

CHAPTER NINE

Entries from my journal

- I don't feel like writing here. I just don't want to have anything to do with the life that I have. I just want it to be easier; I want to run away from it. I feel too numb to express here. I tide through the day somehow. Forcing myself through the unavoidable components, cutting corners, retreating to cry, venting out to husband or family and friends, all the while knowing it will end, and a better day will come.

- Writing twice in one day... feeling very deeply today... sadness and dullness and pain in body. Parents went on a short holiday today. How they take suggestions from me on where to stay, what to order, where to eat, and what to visit, it leaves me so warm and tender inside.

- Today I feel so lonely, so cut off from the people closest to me. All I can feel is my pain and my desperation to escape it. I want to give up and not be judged for it. I feel stuck in the body that has been carrying me for so long because it shows signs of illness despite me pushing myself to keep it healthy...or rather to repair it. Carrying on seems like a punishment. Multiple practitioners to follow up with, to keep treatments coordinated, to reconsider dosages, to reopen closed chapters, to investigate causes...it is endless pain and I just want it all to end.

- Last week was all about drowning and coming back to the surface with doctors' help. Everything had been flaring up for some time – uctd + heavy periods + depression, eventually I wanted it all to end. But this has not happened for the first time. I have been here before. The gap increases a lot each time. That's my victory! I did not give up. I kept fighting and I am still here to write. The writing is laboured. I can't focus.

- Periods come to slow us down. But when you are already going slow, they can make you stop. I have decided that I will neither wait for them nor stop my life when they arrive. I will simply take medicines to check the discomfort and then keep going. I can't afford the impact on my system and routine. It takes away all my power. I can't give it any more. I will continue to do the things I do, on daily basis, rather than resting during periods. At least, I will not lie down. Sitting is ok but no resting. I will keep on moving around in the house and even outside as much as possible. For crochet, I can use sitting posture but I will keep taking breaks to move around. Let's see how it goes this time.

- Last few days were about carrying out my medication + meditation + breathing routine to sustain me through the arthritis flare up. A difficult period plus fever and pains didn't leave me for a clear head to write here. But what I have learnt is that consistency in this routine is all I can manage and exactly what I need. Everything else will have to wait.

- Around the PMS week, my mind gives up on me, or rather takes over from me. I become weepy, anxious, insecure, victim-like and get mental fog. I become disinterested in work and other activities that are absolutely essential for my mental and physical health. I question everything. I resent the people I live with and love. What is most bothersome is that I forget about the things that can soothe me, like crochet, Netflix, talking to mom. By the time I remember, I have already suffered so much.

- I am in a pool of tears. I feel this is an aberration in an otherwise energetic day that I am having today after a long haul of feeling low. I will bounce back today.

- After so many tough days, today, I didn't constantly break down. I was less irritable and impatient. I want to say I am very grateful for the love, support and wonder that is my life. That includes me, my will to get better and the people in my life, especially my parents, husband, my doctor and my therapist.

- Today, I will sketch here, am a little distracted, so I don't feel like writing. I want to enjoy instead. I want to do the pending self-care chores for the rest of the evening. I want to watch some tv as well. Sketch of bird using circles, semi-circle, triangles etc. This is how I draw a bird. This is something I learnt in Nigeria (childhood) and it's my go-to sketch always.

- Last time I was here, I doodled. It made me feel lighter. I am returning after a week. This past week was a reminder that no matter how tough I find my life, I have to independently support myself for physical, moral and emotional support.

Disclaimer

This book is meant to be read as Nishtha's reflection on her journey, not as a reflection on or of the professional advice of any mental health practitioner.